Disclaimer

Vickie Gould is not a medical doctor. This book is not intended to diagnose, treat, cure or prevent any disease. This book is not intended as medical advice. This book is only intended to share Vickie Gould's personal experiences in her own health journey. This book is provided for informational and educational purposes only, not as a treatment guide or instructions for any disease.

Many disease are serious and requires the treatment of a licensed physician. This book is not to be used to substitute for professional medical care. Do not begin any new treatment program without full consent and supervision from a licensed physician. If you have a medical problem, consult a doctor, not this book. If you are pregnant or breastfeeding, consult a doctor before using any treatment.

Vickie Gould offers no guarantee that the ideas in this book are the best therapies for your condition(s). They are simply ideas that the author felt compelled to write about. Do not rely on this book as final treatment in any condition however mild or severe.

☐

I dedicate this book to my children. It is only because of them that I am still here today.

Table of Contents

Forward

I don't want anyone to suffer like I have. I want to help everyone live the life they were meant for. These days, I wake up looking forward to things rather than dreading them. I have hopes and dreams and things I want to do beyond the next hour. I can schedule things now AND show up!

You know - our bodies have this innate ability to try to be well. It constantly, daily fights off pathogens that we don't even notice. It's constantly trying to get to balance, or homeostatis. This is that sweet spot in our health where we feel GOOD. When everything inside is working right, our body normalizes itself and we have energy, sleep well, react to stress well and maintain our ideal weight without much effort. Life is good then.

Hindsight is 20-20 right? I see in retrospect that for me, the dots really do connect if I lay them out in front of me. And I'm going to show you how these can connect for you too. Your Aha! moment is coming up!

Vickie Gould, Master Herbalist, Health and Wellness Coach,
creator of the Release Your Abundant Life Formula

Preface

"My life is over," I think. "I can manage this way for the rest of my life," I try to convince myself for the 1,000th time. "It will be ok if I'm like this forever," I remind myself. I keep trying to let go of the life I used to have and the life I thought I would have in the future. I try to tell myself I'm lucky I got sick in my mid 30's. At least I had some good times in life to look back on. I just wish I felt like I had some to look forward to as well.

I can remember back to two distinct times in my life that seem to have changed the course of my health. The first is during one of our family's moves and a new job for me. My husband and I both got really sick. He got better and I did too eventually, but I never felt the same afterwards. The second is after a very stressful business order (at the time I was making artisan jewelry) and BAM! I can't move my hand, my pain is skyrocketing and it's really hard to function anymore.

I spend my days with migraines, stiff neck and back, fatigue, anger, depression, insomnia, constipation and skin problems. I look at my kids and wish I could be a better, more active mom. I'm missing their childhood. I can't enjoy them growing up. I can't play with them. I can't even muster up the energy to bake cupcakes for their birthday for school, much less go to a party or field trip. I used to never miss those. Who have I become? Where is my life?

I don't understand why doctors can't figure me out. They say I'm fine but I know something's wrong. I can't even get up off the couch to get a sippy cup for my youngest son. It is too much work. It takes too much energy.

Finally, one doctor tells me I have lupus. He wants to give me drugs, but I just don't feel right about the diagnosis. Second opinions, 3rd opinions. Is it early onset arthritis? Early onset perimenopause? Fibromyaglia? Chronic Fatigue? IBS?

A friend of mine tells me to check out her doctor because I'm just not feeling right about the other doctors. Finally, the right diagnosis, one that actually makes sense. I have Chronic Lyme Disease. I figure that's great, I have a name which means I have a way to get better. I couldn't have been more wrong. I didn't know at the time that chronic Lyme disease is one of the most misunderstood diseases out there. It's not recognized, there's no set protocol, people don't believe you're really sick (doctors too), and insurance doesn't recognize it as a long term illness.

I am spending so many nights on the bathroom floor, sobbing and wishing the pain – physical and emotional would go away. No one understands. I'm a shell of the person I used to be. I don't even recognize myself anymore. I feel worthless as a mom, as a wife and as a person.

My husband and I are fighting all the time. I'm angry all the time. My sister asks why I am so angry every time we talk. I don't even know how to answer. I don't go to any social activities anymore. Can't barely drive my kids to school. I get lost in the parking lot of the grocery store.

I feel like my intellect is gone. The brain fog and fatigue is overwhelming. I can't find the right words anymore, I can't do simple math anymore. I can't concentrate on anything for any length of time and I can't follow a conversation, especially if I'm upset. My pride was my intelligence. I loved how much I used to be able to do for my family and others. My worth is dwindling down to nothing. To top it off, my husband wants to leave me. This is the bottom of my deep black hole.

I start bargaining with God to take me now. I don't understand – Am I being punished for something I did? Please Lord, just let me die. I think up ways to end it, but I don't want to traumatize whoever has to find me.

Then I bargain with God to please make me better instead because I can't bear for my children to grow up without a mother, even one as useless as me. But it doesn't happen and I'm back to trying to convince myself to be ok with this for the rest of my life. I just can't though. So I go numb instead.

Honestly, what I really want is to be normal again and have my life back. I want energy; I want to stop feeling numb. I'm tired, really tired of what my life has amounted to and of who I've become and I don't know what to do anymore. What I'm saying to myself in my head isn't working at all.

Doctors are useless. They don't know what to do with me. I'm "too complex". What am I going to do? I want answers. I want to get to the root problem. Why am I not getting better? Is this really my destiny?

Years are passing me by. My kids are growing up. I've given up so much. I've missed so much. I am bitter.

I want to just enjoy one sunny day, with enough stamina to last. Is that too much to ask?

Crying every night is getting old and making my eyes puffy and giving me headaches. My heart feels literally like it's going to pound out of my chest and explode. What are my choices? What can I do?

I know now it's my time to do it on my own and give the fight of my life, for my life. I've plateaued. I'm not getting better. I can either choose to keep sobbing every night or I can choose to do something about it. I'm only 40 and I should have 40-50 more years to go, right? I can't imagine 40 years of this torture, so the only other thing to do is figure it out myself.

Along the way, I've been reading up on alternative healing methods, nutrition, herbs and supplements. I'm learning about how the body works and all the people I've talked to who are in my same boat are researching for themselves too. It's during this time I decide to become a Master Herbalist so that when I'm done, I can help others too.

During this time I also find a great nurse practitioner and she teaches me about hormone balancing and mold toxicity. Of course, I go off and learn more on my own because that's just how I am. What a blessing she has been!

Hallelujah, the light is on at the end of the tunnel! One day I notice that I don't have to take naps throughout my day. Another day I realize that the activities I did the day before, haven't done me in for the next day. Then I notice that my mood is lifting, I'm scheduling things and looking forward to activities. Wow, what a difference! I have ME back! My husband notices too (and yes, we have our happy forever after).

I know now you're wondering what I did that turned my bleak destiny around and I promise I'm going to share those discoveries with you in the next pages. So hold on to your seats and get ready to discover YOU again. Life on the other side is so much better!

Introduction

I don't know why you've picked up this book today, but I want you to know that I care about you. I want you to know that you're not alone. Whether you're here for general health issues, chronic issues or even some serious issues, I challenge you to keep an open mind about what I'm going to tell you and implement these strategies not only with yourself but with your family. Right now is a great opportunity for you to transform your life and change so that you don't have to deal with your health problems forever.

I'm sure you've heard of people who have overcome "incurable" diseases or overcome obstacles to walk again after being paralyzed, baffling conventional medicine. In the words of Christopher Reeve - So many of our dreams at first seem impossible, then they seem improbable and then when we summon the will, they soon become inevitable". If you've been told that you have to "live with it" for the rest of your life, are you willing to trust that they're right and there's no way to feel better?

It's no secret there's a health crisis in America. If you notice, people are more and more sluggish and overweight. They are depressed, suffer from chronic illness, aches, pains, headaches and brain fog. On top of it, they just look sad. More and more pharma is being handed out like candy. But have you ever wondered - do you really think that your body deficiency is a pharma drug?

Your body is very intelligent and we don't seem to give it enough credit. All day long it is trying to tell you what it needs and internally it is trying to keep everything in balance. So if you have high sugar, your body will produce hormones to try to reduce it. If you have too much stress, your body will try to produce hormones to block it. And on the simplest level, if you need water, it will make you feel thirsty. If we can tune in and try to understand the signals better, we can answer with the right response.

We also live with a lot of pollutants –things that you don't even think about. Your antibacterial hand soap is an endocrine disruptor. Soy increases your estrogen. The perfume that the lady next to you is wearing is toxic to your body. The chlorine in your pool water can be toxic too. The normal fumes that you encounter outside from lawn mowers, cars or trucks affect your body in ways you may never have really thought about. What about the pesticides on your lawn, not to mention in your food?

With all these stressors, it's no wonder you're feeling sluggish and foggy.

How can you expect to be energetic or "with it"?

But you don't have to feel like there's no hope because there are answers. You just need to know what they are!

I have been health coaching for a number of years now and I want to tell you how much it saddens me to see people who feel stuck in a rut or frozen in their current situation. I am here to tell you that it isn't necessary! Don't "settle" for a mundane life. Have the life you were meant to live! We all have a purpose here and our purpose is not to just "get by". Each of us has something to contribute to the world.

Imagine your life 1 year from now, 2 years from now, 5 years from now. Wouldn't it be nice if you could .....

Get a refreshing night's sleep?
Stop feeling overwhelmed?
Sparkle from happiness inside?
Feel Ninja - like you could conquer anything?
Manage your stress well?
Have a passion and a zeal for your life?
Add pleasure, contentment and satisfaction to your life?

Get ready to feel alive! Get ready to feel joy, passion, pleasure, happiness, peace and contentment. When you take ownership of your future, you'll be more fulfilled, your family life will be better and you'll actually be completely participating in your life - with zest!

Your friends are seriously going to ask you what you did - Can you imagine the things you could accomplish?

This is all YOU now. You must be ready and eager to learn and want to feel better. We have to take back the responsibility of our health from our doctors to ourselves. We need to be our own advocates. This is the only way to combat the chronic issues plaguing people today. YOU are in charge of your destiny..... and I think it's looking pretty good from here!

Release Your Abundant Life Formula program is no longer available.

Background

Until I got sick with Lyme and my mistrust grew with our medical system, I didn't question what I was being told by the medical community. I thought the CDC, FDA, pharma manufacturers were all here for my benefit. After all, we all really want to believe that the systems created for us are actually for us, but they're not.

The basis of being healthy is allowing your body to do what it naturally wants to do. Each day it fights invisible things that can be tiny attacks on our well-being. Most of the time it does fine with it, but when things pile up on top of each other, our body loses its ability to function properly. With as poisonous as today's lives are -- environmentally and emotionally, sometimes our bodies need a little help. We give it help by clearing out things that get in the way. What are those things that get in the way of our physical bodies? Poisons – Toxins!

I know you probably struggle with a lot of the same symptoms I did and my clients do – lack of energy, constant fatigue, weight gain, insomnia, brain fog, allergies and sensitivities, skin problems and digestive issues.

In your old way of doing things, you may have tried:
- Coffee and energy drinks
- Sleeping pills
- Bootcamp exercising
- Go with the fads
- Endless spinning your wheels

- Frustration that leads to giving up
- Not being able to keep on track
- Searching the internet for contrary information or ask friends

In the new way of doing things, you're going to understand why your body may be reacting the way it is, learn to understand what it's trying to tell you and also figure out what you can do to help it get back to optimum performance. After all, this is what you want right? Then you'll be able to get back to your regularly scheduled life, with energy and zest. The only way you'll succeed is to commit to the education process and take positive action toward reaching your goals.

During my search, my question was always "What is it about a person that makes them more susceptible to something, given the same exposure as someone else?" It seems some people recover and others never do. I've spoken to many people who deal with chronic issues and one thing seems prevalent. Their bodies were in prime condition, with multiple layers of issues that made it hard for them to overcome their symptoms. This is the basis of the Release Your Abundant Life Formula program that I created to help people to optimize their bodies so they can have energy, zest and live the life they were meant for.

Everyone I've spoken to seems to have these issues:
- Prime Body Conditions
- Inability to Detox Properly
- Other Chronic Pathogens
- Past Trauma (emotional or physical)

We are constantly dealing with toxic overload from their environment, home and food. These toxins led to food and chemical and environmental sensitivities. We also deal with high levels of inflammation caused by those toxins that sometimes are hidden inside our bodies. The inflammation causes aches and pains and fatigue. That inflammation distracts our bodies from being able to deal with anything else and that leads to poor immune function where it's either overworked and overreacting or the immune system was so tired that it couldn't even mount up a fight to a real threat.

Additionally, people have poor digestion in general. We've all heard that your immune system is in your gut - it's your second brain. With poor digestion comes poor absorption and poor nutrition and poor elimination. These all contribute to chronic fatigue, IBS, fibromyalgia and brain fog to name a few.

In order to reduce the chronic issues, we have to decrease the load the body is taking on with the toxins, inflammation, poor immune function and poor digestion. We need to clear all of it out so that the body can us its own innate ability to be well and live well. By doing this, we rebalance our insides into peak performance.

Sadly, our ability to detox can be hindered by a fairly common gene mutation. Since testing for mutations is somewhat rare, this means that much of the world is walking around with mutations, unbeknownst to them. No wonder 90 million people are estimated to have chronic health problems. When this gene mutation is expressing or turned on, we are unable to properly detox as our bodies should do by itself each day.

Somewhat connected to our inability to detox is the existence of chronic pathogens – for me it was coinfections of Lyme, past problems with strep that reactivated and mold toxicity. You may have some others as well. When these pathogens layer up on top of each other they compound our problems of trying to get better. We need to kill off these chronic pathogens and then detox to get them out of our bodies. This will lessen our body's stress load and lead to feeling better. You will literally feel relieved!

The last thing that people tend to consider in their health hurdles is the effects of trauma on their overall wellness. Many of us have big things that have happened – things from childhood, past relationships, emotional traumas, physical traumas including a sickness, abuse or and accident that hinder our well-being on a daily basis. Many of these things we don't even realize are in our way. Learning to neutralize the effects of these stressors on our lives will help to alleviate our symptoms.

I look for balance, I do not call anything a cure or remission. Many pathogens, viruses, bacteria, etc. stay in your body, but it's when they take over that you have chronic problems. When in balance, your body can keep all these things at bay and you can still feel well, function well and live the life you know you were meant for.

Toxins: Those Pesky Buggers that Steal our Energy

So let's talk more about toxins. At the root of basically all health issues is issues with toxins which are poisons that float around in the air, water, food, etc. It's all around us. Issues with toxins translates into issues with detoxing. In a nutshell, when you have too many toxins going in and not enough getting flushed, out, you get backed up and symptoms or illness happens. Whether you are bombarded with a lot of toxins like a huge wave or waterfall and it puts you over or if it's a little drip each day that builds up over time but never gets flushed out fast enough, this excess of toxins floating around in your body causes people a lot of problems. Think of each toxin as having spears and swords and as they float through our bloodstream and body, it's piercing the blood vessels and organs that it passes by. As time goes on, these injuries add up.

Our world has become more toxic through the years. This issue wasn't nearly as prevalent long ago as it is now. Advances in industry and science has contributed to the pollution in our air, water and food.

Basically if you're living and breathing, you have toxicity. They're now saying from the Columbia University School of Public Health that over 95% of cancers are due to our environment. What does this mean for us? What it really means is that everyone has room for improvement. There are some things we can't control, but what we can, we should.

These days, so many of us have symptoms of toxin overload - which equates to a body system overload. Many have system related disease - autoimmune, cancer, MS, ALS, colitis, skin conditions, mental disorders, celiac, GERD, allergies - every disease is directly or indirectly related to toxins. You wake up unrefreshed, don't sleep well, have insomnia, chronic fatigue, brain fog, lowered stamina, have bad breath and body odor, dark circles under your eyes, minor and major aches and pains, bowel problems/ IBS, hair loss, skin discoloration, depression, anxiety, etc.

Health for us in this century is getting more and more elusive and problems are starting younger and younger. Babies are now being born with toxin overload inherited from mom. We've all heard that babies get their mother's immune system, well, that also includes their gut flora, which is their gut health, their nutrient deficiencies and then also their toxins. Cord blood studied by the EWG (Environmental Working Group) showed that newborns begin life exposed to 257 of 413 toxic chemicals studied. The average is 200 toxins found per baby and 101 toxins found in ALL babies. (a healthy adult has 90 toxins). Then start shooting in toxic vaccines and then what do you think happens.... but that's a whole huge other topic.

Dr. Russell Blaylock, a neuroscientist said, "Unfortunately, I predict disaster in the next 20 years for today's children who are so widely and intensely affected now by toxins that when they reach 30 and 40, they are going to be sick and dying.... in much greater numbers than today. So I pray that people start paying attention."

So where do these toxins come from? They come from our indoor and outdoor air, water, food - low fat, processed, sugar filled foods, food dyes, chemicals in household cleaners, pesticides we use on our lawn and flowerbeds, chemicals in our laundry detergent, body and skincare items, deodorant, perfumes, toothpaste, plastics used in everyday living, EMFs, toxic gasses coming off our carpet, beds and furniture, "new car" smell, over the counter and prescription medicines - so many and too many to keep listing. We are assaulted every day. We need to know what to throw back at it.

But we've been lied to. We're told that pharmaceuticals are what our bodies need, but do you really thing that our bodies are deficient in some chemical like that? We've been told food additives are "safe", lawn products and Monsanto's roundup is "safe" and GMO's are "safe". We've been told everything in moderation, but if you understand the tipping point that toxins create, you'll know that moderation is still going to make the toxins overflow faster than we can get it out. It is absolutely NOT safe at all. And to compound the problem, a weak toxin + another weak toxin can = a large synergistic toxin which has a much much bigger effect on our lives than the little ones alone.

The human body is fascinating. We don't even yet know everything that it can do, but its ability to heal and self-regulate is beyond what we are led to believe. We need to use ourselves FOR ourselves rather that looking outside for help. Inside is truly what counts!

The problem with toxins is that they accumulate. Studies show that the level of one of the toxins, pesticides, in people's blood correspond to age, not weight - the people who are the oldest have the most pesticides in their blood. Because there are so many sources, our bodies can get bogged down and backed up and can't keep up. So we get more toxins in than we can flush out per day. Some people have extra issues like gene mutations that make it even more difficult. But we can address that too. So it's ALL OK! Awareness and education really does claim the day. Also, studies have shown that those who attack this with a buddy, TOGETHER as we do in Release Your Abundant Life Formula have twice as much success as those who try to do it alone.

So what can do we do to get rid of the toxins? We detoxify our bodies. But before we detox, we have to prep because if our bodies aren't ready to receive the help, it not work well at all.

The Foundation: Preparing Yourself to Be Well

Honestly, I was tempted to skip this part for fear of overloading you and as we say "puking on your shoes" with information. But I just couldn't reconcile if you were to go out and detox with this step, it would fail because your body isn't prepared to accept the detox process. I'm hoping that you can handle all the info that you're about to get.

First we need to look at prepping your kitchen:

We can't go into everything about food and nutrition here (this is actually a whole multi-step module in the Release your Abundant Life Formula), but what I want to tell you is that if you never change your food, you will never be well. By ingesting poisons every day, you add to your body's burden.

If you've never heard of Genetically Modified Organisms (food), then you should look it up. Created by poison giant, Monsanto, the same company that created Agent Orange. That in itself doesn't make sense. Why would the company that made Agent Orange be part of our food supply? Just think about that a moment and you'll see it just doesn't make sense. GMO's were never meant to be in our food supply. If you investigate the history of Monsanto, you'll see that this is NOT good for us. GMO's have been shown to cause cancer, yet it's still on our grocery shelves as are things like aspartame, food dyes, MSG, and other chemicals that are banned in other countries - there's a reason for that!! The US really needs to get on board!

So the best thing to do is eat organic foods, non GMO's - make sure you know the clean 15 and the dirty dozen lists so you can make informed decisions on which foods may be ok non-organic. (Hint: cross reference these lists because some of the produce with the least pesticides are that way because they are GMO) And make sure you ditch the processed foods, fast foods and junk food, especially sugar of any kind. Please do not tell me that the cost of organics is too high. The cost of illness is much much much higher and the cost of losing your quality of life or your entire life is even higher. You're here because you want your life back right? You won't get it by staying where you are, eating the same garbage and hoping it doesn't have as much of an affect as I'm saying it does. Trust me, it definitely has that much of an affect!!

Please also be aware and willing to eliminate the top food intolerances that cause toxin overload and inflammation and be aware these could be your culprits. The top ones are: wheat/gluten, dairy, sugar, corn, soy, eggs, yeast, tree nuts, fish and shellfish, peanuts. An Elimination Diet (also laid out in Release Your Abundant Life Formula) is crucial to finding out which foods are your personal culprits for some of your symptoms such as bloating, constipation or diarrhea, weight gain, headaches, inflammation, brain fog, sleep issues, fatigue, autoimmune diseases and joint pain. This can also affect your hormones!

If it were up to me, none of us would ever eat wheat, dairy or white sugar. These are all highly inflammatory. I cannot tell you how many people I know who just with that step have increased their energy, decreased their brain fog and fixed digestive issues. As Hippocrates said "All diseases begin in the stomach"

A side note to wheat/gluten - It's not our grandparents' wheat. It's been morphed and hybridized. Just go check out old photos of wheat. It doesn't even look the same anymore. No single dietary protein is a more potent trigger of neuro dysfunction and neuro autoimmunity than gluten, the protein in wheat. Immense reactions to gluten can break down the blood brain barrier and causes severe inflammatory reactions in people. Those facts alone should send you screaming in the other direction from wheat.

I could go on about sugar in much the same way as wheat/gluten. The average toddler has consumed as much sugar already in their short life as our grandparents did their whole entire lives. Sugar is toxic, plain and simple, even organic sugar causes inflammation.

During your health journey, you may need to also address food addictions and attitudes that could hold you back from moving forward.

Be warned when you prep your kitchen and pantry, you will be throwing out food (and the frugal person in me cringes at this like you do) -- I know it stinks, but it's worth it. Cooking is going to become your ally and snacks like carrot sticks and grapes or strawberries will be your friends. As Dr. Mark Hyman says, "Your health depends on cooking and our survival depends on health."

Next, it's good to understand how important our air and water is really is. When everything that's attacking us is invisible, it's hard to really "get" how critical it is or even take it seriously. 95% of toxicants in our homes are bound to carpet, dust, fabrics, upholstery and drapery. Our air really bombards us, especially when lawn pesticides are sprayed or farmers spray their crops. Car and truck fumes pass us by every day too.

It has been studied all over the world that when outdoor pollution increases, more people show up at emergency rooms with heart attacks. And the indoor air in our home contains mold spores and contaminants from cleaning. Get a heavy duty air filter for your home air duct system and clean the ducts out if possible. Use high quality air filters and change more often. Open windows if the outside air quality is better. Live houseplants can help (watch you don't mold the soil).

Many people seem to like to wear strong perfume, use air fresheners at work, at home and in the car. The problem with this is that the fumes are toxic. They can even be carcinogenic. If you breathe that in every day, what do you think is happening, especially if you're not working on detoxing each day? Those toxins will get stored in your body, recirculated and may even be contributing to that excess weight you're trying to lose!

Make sure your basement is clear of fumes and moisture too. Poor quality air is one of the top 5 environmental risks. Think your home is safe? Think again. 54% more women who work at home get cancer and this is due to the chemicals in household products. Cleaning products are the 3rd most common reason for exposures to poison in adults. UGH!

Many toxins are clearly associated with obesity and type 2 diabetes -- both which are obviously on the rise in our country.

Don't forget your water holds many chemical assailants too. Most municipalities' water is contaminated with recycled sewage, traces of chemicals and medications go into the water from humans and animals. All meds end up in groundwater and chlorine, chloramine, fluoride is in our water. Get a good filter like a Berkey Water Filter for your water to take out chlorine, fluoride, and heavy metals. Drink alkaline water when you can. You can simply add lemon to your water and it will help you detox. You can choose to use Reverse Osmosis filtering but it takes out too much, and you'll need to re-mineralize afterwards. If you buy water, use spring water only.

Last but not least, you also have to prep your mind for being well because wanting to be well and committing to be well are 2 different things. Sometimes we hang on to what is "comfortable" and "known" even if it's bad and we don't want it because what we don't know is seems scarier. To get healthy, you have to have an attitude of no excuses and no procrastination. You've got to be done with the low energy, low happiness life you have and commit to succeeding in getting the life you want.

Success is not a goal or a wish or desire. It's a commitment to succeed and not let anything get in your way, including nay-sayers (those in your head too).

You must get ready to take action and change your life and lifestyle. You must be ok with being uncomfortable and struggling. You must be ready to take in knowledge and put it to use. It's best to align your mind with your intentions and go after it with a vengeance. People who want to be a part of Release Your Abundant Life are only accepted to the program if they are 110% committed and doing this for themselves (not their spouse, kids, mom or dad). Getting well is going to take effort and time. You didn't get to where you are overnight and it won't change overnight either. Steady wins the race.

Detox: Getting Rid of the Monsters Inside of You

Our bodies were designed to detox daily. If we didn't naturally detox at all, then we would die. When you have chronic issues, detoxing more is really important, but it may also take a while to finish it all up and get things moving along right again. Some people may feel a little worse before they get better, especially if you're really overly toxic but never fear, that feeling should go away in a few days. A journal of what you're doing, what you're experiencing and how you're feeling physically and emotionally can help you along your health journey.

How do you detox correctly to get rid of the toxins? You must fix your toxin load at the cellular level, in your colon/digestive tract and in your liver.

Cellular level is important and many forget this, but the cell membrane needs to stay soft and flexible so there is proper fluid exchange. You need potassium to pull waste out and sodium to drive nutrients in. You are only going to be as healthy as your cells are. How do you help your cells? Simply by using good healthy fats which we'll talk about in a little bit.

Now let me say that if you already know your greatest exposure to toxins, STOP IT! Decrease your toxins going in and increase your toxins going out. This is how you get to feeling right again.

There are many of us who have a harder time detoxing than others. Probably 50% of the population has a gene mutation called MTHFR (yes I know what it looks like) and it keeps us from detoxing well. If you're having issues with the symptoms I've already mentioned (which is probably why you're here), I'd bet you're one of us mutants.

The guts and the liver are two detox organs that are super important and the focus of what we are going to start detoxing here. They are not all inclusive in the process, but extremely important. You must get these 2 things running smoothly in order to have detox be successful. The biggest body energy expenditure is in digestion so we need to make digestion as easy as possible for us to conserve that energy.

But first, we can't talk about detox without talking about inflammation. Toxins cause inflammation, food intolerances cause inflammation, breathing toxins cause inflammation and inflammation throughout the body causes pain and health issues. How do you think your brain functions when it's swollen and inflamed? There's a direct path from your guts to your brain and when your guts are inflamed, your brain is inflamed. How do you think your joints feel when they're inflamed? Have you ever noticed sometimes your face is puffy or your feet feel swollen? There's dark puffy circles under your eyes - that's inflammation. You absolutely cannot be healthy if your guts are inflamed and that's mostly caused by toxins.

Toxins can also cause what's called leaky gut. Leaky gut happens when the lining of the intestines get small holes - remember those toxins with spears and swords? There's supposed to be a mucus lining protecting the gut walls which is your immune system, but it gets damaged with toxins. Good fats from things like Omega 3's like avocados, nuts, grass fed beef help line the gut and protect it from toxins. Good fats heal and seal. When toxins overtake the guts, the lining gets small holes that allow the toxins to go back into the bloodstream causing retoxification -- those pesky toxins just cut in line and got a free ride back through your body! What other things leak back through the lining? Bacteria, Viruses, parasites and food particles -- all these things were on the way OUT and now they've been let back in. It's pretty easy to see why this is a big compounding problem now. Leaky gut can also cause bloating, food sensitivities, thyroid issues, brain fog, digestive issues, headaches, joint pain and more inflammation. It's a vicious cycle.

By the time you experience noticeable symptoms, your liver is on overload, not just your guts. The liver performs over 1,000 daily tasks and is often overlooked and forgotten in health but it filters every drop of blood that flows through it. It produces chemicals to combat viruses and bacteria along with antihistamines to neutralize things that promote the growth of cancer. 80% of your liver can be damaged before you ever have any symptoms! According to Dr. Kasper Bond who wrote The Liver and Cancer, "No disease, especially degenerative diseases including cancer and AIDS could survive longer than a few weeks in the presence of a healthy liver." Let's let that sink in for a minute and think about the fact that basically everyone has a sluggish liver these days.

Once the liver is overburdened, it passes on the burden to the kidneys and that causes chronic low back pain, sweaty palms, bags under the eyes, frequent urination, and bladder infections. Then when the kidneys can't hold on any longer, it passes the burden to the bladder, then the lymph system..... but all that's more than what we can cover here. Bottom line is if your liver isn't functioning at optimum, you will never feel good.

We've already talked about cleaning up your food and environment. Now we need to talk about how to clean up the mess inside our bodies. So to start, I like to clean out the guts so we can get the gut flora right again. According to Dr. Mercola, "The interconnectedness of your gut, brain, immune and hormonal systems is impossible to unwind. The past few years have brought a scientific flurry of information about how crucial your microflora are to your genetic expression, immune system, body weight and composition, mental health, memory and minimizing your risk for numerous diseases."

Everyone could use some help in their colon. If your digestive tract isn't working, nothing is working. Colon is the repository for oxidative stress, abnormal fermentation (like putrification) and is really a battleground. Many have issues with absorption in the small intestine but it's harder to fix if your large intestine/colon is messed up. And when the absorption doesn't work right, you end up reabsorbing the toxins into your body and the toxins are recirculated creating that retoxification that daily increases your toxin load.

There's a really easy way to clean out your guts with vitamin C (if your stomach is sensitive, then use ester-C). Take 1000 mg every 1/2 -1 hour until you poop like tapioca. Definitely do this on a day that you're going to be home all day. Don't use not having a free day as an excuse not to do this step. Other things you can use to clean out your guts are psyllium husk, flax, and pectin.

To additionally help improve your bowel elimination process:
1. Increase hydration
2. Add good fats

3.   Use high quality probiotics
4.   Increase fiber

Sometimes those toxins need to be dragged kicking and screaming out of your body. You can use binders to do that. The toxins will stick to the binder and the binder is then expelled by your body through your poop (I'm a mom, so I use these technical terms). My favorite binder is diatomaceous earth because it's easy to take, doesn't bind to the good stuff and can also kill parasites in your intestinal tract as it flows through. There are other good binders like activated charcoal, bentonite clay, and chlorella.

Like I mentioned before, healthy fats create that protective barrier our intestines need to help flush out viruses, bacteria, parasites, fungi, toxins and other pathogens our body is trying to get rid of. Increase your healthy fats and clean supplements. No fats in the diet causes brain shrinkage and then the toxins in your brain have extra room to stay and get cozy.

Our guts can be laid out the length of a tennis court and it contains about 3.5 to 5 pounds of beneficial bacteria. The good and bad bacteria divide and multiply every 20 minutes. What's the purpose of all this bacteria? That good bacteria synthesizes nutrients like vitamin B necessary for energy and helps metabolize nutrients like proteins, fats and carbs so our bodies get what it needs. You can see why having more of the good guys to outnumber the bad guys really matters! It's really important to take a high quality probiotic to get your soldiers lined up in there.

Additionally, your guts create 95% of the serotonin (the happy hormone) your body needs. When your flora is unbalanced, you can suffer mood issues. Recent studies have shown that probiotics are a good line of defense with people suffering from depression.

Our national overuse of antibiotics and other meds have created an epidemic of people with bad guts - few of us in this century are walking around with good "normal" gut bacteria. If you have a coated tongue, bad breath, extra vaginal discharge, joint pain, puffiness in your body, or digestive issues, it could be an indication that your gut flora is way out of whack (this can be what's called candida). Additionally, when you have an unbalanced immune system, you lose the ability to fight off viruses and bacteria. You can end up with chronic infections along with a compromised GI tract.

In order to help with the gut flora, along with the high count good probiotics, I like to use things to lower the bad bacteria count. You can use something as simple as coconut oil or things derived from coconut oil like caprylic acid or monolaurin. These will cut down on the candida yeast overgrowth. I also really like grapefruit seed extract except that this can sometimes lower the good bacteria too. I take the grapefruit seed extract first thing in the morning for this reason because I take my probiotics at night.

Because our liver and pancreas are connected, we often need help with a pancreatic enzyme. Take something with amylases, lipases and potcolytic enzymes. When you take it with meals, it's digestive support. When you take it on an empty stomach, it can kill cancer cells. As we age, we naturally, make less of these enzymes and this is why it's important to supplement.

Other things that help the liver are avocado, potassium, gentle fiber, magnesium, fruits and veggies, herb like milk thistle, burdock, dandelion root, parsley, cilantro, oregano, bitter greens, cruciferous veggies, sprouts, and watercress (I wish I liked them). Fermented veggies you make at home are also great and fermented Sulphur foods like garlic and onions may help too. Some people who have candida issues don't do well on fermented foods so just let your body tell you if it enjoys them.

Other things that I love to use for detox include the lemon water I mentioned before, milk thistle herb (or you can get a detox tea), curcumin/turmeric (get only 95% curcuminoids), and epsom salt baths (use 2 cups epsom salt, 1 cup baking soda and 1 ounce 35% food grade hydrogen peroxide – don't drink this straight or get it on your hands because it will burn).

The hydrogen peroxide soaks into your pores and into your blood plasma and oxygenates it. Pathogens like bacteria, parasites, viruses don't like oxygenated environments. In fact it can kill them! This is a great way to help those muscle aches (magnesium) and help rid our bodies of yuck (hydrogen peroxide). And the bonus is, that it is also a stress reliever.

I love to also use essential oils on my feet after my bath. Make sure to mix essential oils with a carrier oil before giving yourself a foot rub. Use a foot reflexology chart for reference if you have trouble spots.

Saunas are awesome for detoxing since the sweat releases toxins. Make sure you wipe down your sauna after use and rinse off your skin too. Instead of sauna, you can use an infrared heat mat (which is what I use). It can also help heal soft tissue.

One very important aspect of detox that is often overlooked and not taken very seriously is sleep. Your liver does most of its filtering during your sleep, so if you don't get enough sleep or your sleep is not deep or it's interrupted regularly, you won't get the full benefit of natural detox. It's simple, but probably the thing that people are most resistant to and could be hard if you have sleep problems caused by health issues. If you're having problems sleeping, I would try valerian root, gaba, magnesium (not oxide because it doesn't absorb well), bach rescue remedies or a sleep tea with lavender and chamomile.

People tell me they're a night owl but we were not made to be night owls. We were made to go to sleep when it got dark and get up when the sun is up. This is your natural circadian rhythm. Those who are night owls are generally backwards because their adrenals are stressed which is another layer of illness that we get into in the Release Your Abundant Life Formula. You really need minimally 7-8 hours of sleep each night but if you're trying to specifically do a detox, if you can increase it to 9-10 hours, you would benefit greatly from it.

Remember I said that some people may have symptoms during detox? Don't worry, they'll pass. But stay the course. Your symptoms may include flu-like symptoms, fatigue, lethargy, headache, joint pain, aches, fevers, rashes (skin is the largest detox organ). You can take a 5 day break and then start up again.

Please keep in mind that with good nutrition and good detox, our amazing bodies can do about anything which means that you can do and be anything you want to be. According to Dr. Crinnion, "If people learn to have a clean home and watch their diets, they could drop the circulating level of toxicants in their bodies by close to 80% within 2-3 weeks."

Let's go over a checklist for detoxing since so much information has been given. This is all laid out for you easily in the Release Your Abundant Life Formula as well.

1. If you know the source of your toxins, STOP it immediately
2. Eat clean and have a chemical free home
3. Clean your colon out with vitamin C
4. Replenish your good gut bacteria with high quality
5. Detox your liver with herbs, saunas, baths and use an enzyme supplement
6. Make getting good sleep a priority

Bottom line is if you can get your body cleaned up with detoxing and add in the good clean nutrients it needs, your body can finally have a chance to improve and heal itself. You'll be free of those symptoms that plague you and you'll have more energy, be in a better mood, and be able participate in your own life again.

Stress: The Invisible Thief Who Steals our Lives

Everyone knows stress is bad for you, but no one seems to know what to do about it. On top of it, I've noticed that people seem to actually brag about how much they have to do or how little sleep they get and how much they have to multitask. They seem to actually like to feel like they're working hard and really overextended with kids' activities. Why is that? Why have we become a society that one –ups each other on how stressed we are? This is not good! I want you to know that taking care of yourself is not selfish or lazy or indulgent; it's medically necessary. If you've ever flown in an airplane before, you remember how they say to take care of your oxygen mask before assisting others. This is life too. You cannot effectively do anything for the ones you love if you let your own health take a backseat to everyone else's needs.

Did you know that the amount of chronic stress people endure is a good predictor of longevity? People who have lower stress, but are obese or smoke may have longer lives than those who do not know how to mitigate stress. Again, this is not good!

Try this exercise: write the numbers 1 through 17 on one line. Underneath it, write "I am not stressed". How long did it take you? How did it feel? Not very stressful, right? Now write both lines, but alternating one number then one letter then one number until you're done. How long did it take? How did you feel? It's kind of stressful isn't it? This is what happens when you're constantly multi-tasking.

What I AM going to share with you today is really near and dear to my heart. You would not believe the amount of people who ask me -- how can I just GET THROUGH my day, my problems, my illness? How can I just survive my day? I'm an emotional wreck.

My heart breaks. I know all too well how it feels to be a burden to your family because you're too sick to function, feel useless and are stressed out trying to fight an illness and have a life - live a life. I want to show you how you can neutralize stress, reframe stressful thoughts and find ways to relax. You are worth taking care of because YOU are worth it.

Right now is your time and your opportunity to transform your life and learn what you can do to take back control of your mind, body and life. How much would it be worth to you to have you again - your life back again? Can you even put a price tag on it? 1,000 dollars? 10,000 dollars? 100,000 dollars? 1 million dollars? Of course not - it's priceless.

What I'm sharing is missing a piece of our health puzzle that's commonly overlooked by doctors. It's the connection that the mind has with our physical well-being. I want to be clear that I'm not talking about it "being all in your head" nor am I talking about "mind over matter". Much the opposite. I want to talk about how the very real stress and past traumas you have in your mind and from outside influences can hinder your attempts to be well.

Listen, I know about this because I lived through this. The only thing that stood in my way was my "want to". I had to muster up my will to go on and keep at it even when I wanted to give up. Each step seemed so hard, but looking back, I'm so glad I took these steps because I'm so happy I've gotten to where I am now.

One of the things that people with chronic illness face is the circular problem that stress creates - past, present, short term and long term. Stress causes flares. Stress causes loss of hope. It becomes this circular thing where stress makes you feel bad, but then you get upset and stressed about stress and it seems like a never ending hole. It keeps you from improving and it makes it really hard to emotionally get through a particular moment or an entire stage of life. I'm going to show you ways you can neutralize and reframe stress today so you can have that amazing life you know you deserve.

Your overall stress load comes from many places - emotional, physical, relationship, environmental, spiritual, work stress, diet stress, survival stress, exercise stress, etc.

They did a study on people and asked them if they viewed stress as bad. Then tracked who died. Those who felt that stress was bad died earlier. What does this mean? Our opinion of what stress does to us may affect how that stress actually affects us. Interesting, huh?

It could be that if you tell your mind that your stress response is your body preparing for something and view that response as helpful, you could offset the "bad" from that stress response. If we can train ourselves to react better in our typical stress response, we may be able to neutralize it. Thinking of our response to stress as courage in a situation may help us get through that situation. Just think about this quote from Peter McWilliams, "Our thoughts create our reality - where we put our focus is the direction we tend to go." We can kindly guide those thoughts so they are more beneficial to our lives.

Your physical and mental responses are connected. Everyone has some level of this connection. Just think about the last time you got embarrassed. Your physical response was your face got red. Or when you're asked to speak in front of 100's of people. Your stomach tightens up. A stressful day may give you a "tension headache". Stress triggers emotions that trigger physical responses and this is very real. Emotions are very powerful indeed and these emotions can cause real physical symptoms such as pain. The emotions of repressed, unresolved or unexpressed anger, sadness or stress can actually give us chronic problems. In fact, sometimes your body creates pain to distract you from your emotional problems so you don't have to deal with them.

Chronic low level (or high level) stress and tension can lead to multiple physical responses. Things like chronic fatigue, IBS, fibromyalgia, chronic back pain can have a mind connection as part of the problem. If there are no structural or biochemical indications, sometimes thinking back to the onset of the emotional turmoil will help pinpoint, then alleviate the issue.

A person's emotional life can point to places and times that caused problems. Stress and tension, pressure and personality are all factors. Many have recurring issues with things that happened when they were young, traumatic events in their lives, family and people they find hard to deal with and work or life situations that seemingly can't be changed. These can all lead to chronic issues continuing since they are going unaddressed and unresolved. Additionally this chronic stress can zap your energy, create insomnia and increase pain. By rethinking, reframing and neutralizing past and present stressors, you may be able help change your physical problems.

In the days of the caveman, we had spurts of energy with adrenaline to go out and hunt for food or defend against an attacker. Our Fight or Flight response kicked in for short amounts of time. Then we slowed down, calmed down, settled in and things were peaceful again. These days, we deal with daily stresses and the Fight or Flight response is all day long. Our baseline of stress is much higher than it was years ago and that means that the adrenaline never stops flowing. This is a problem. Our bodies were never meant to release adrenaline all day long. This can cause a bunch of health issues. And without getting too technical with cortisol and the adrenal glands and all the other endocrine glands it effects, just know that this constant stress wears our bodies out. We go into this in much more detail in Release Your Abundant Life Formula if you want to know more.

As Dr. Alan Christianson says, "Life is like a 4 burner stove". Each burner is Family, Friends, Health and Work. It's very hard to have all 4 burners going at the same time. Most people can't do this. You can really only have 2 going per day and be successful.

Stress can be defined as anything that triggers survival mode (Fight or Flight). Stress can come from those things already listed and also dietary stress, physical stress including exercise, mental stress and environmental stress. Some of those stressors were discussed in the topics relating to toxins and detoxing. I'm going to show you how to deal with emotional stresses and how to neutralize them so that they don't create physical problems too. People who live a thriving, abundant life do not live a stress free life, they've just learned to overcome their stressors so there's less of an impact.

Hans Seyle, in 1936, identified the 3 stages of stress: alarm (stress identified), resistance (when the body attempts to cope with the stress), and exhaustion (when the body's resources are depleted, functioning is no longer normal and long-term damage can occur).

Chronic stress has been shown to impair growth and development and lead to metabolic, immune, hormonal and psychiatric disorders. During certain times in your life like periods in the womb (yes, even before you're born), infancy, childhood or adolescence, neural pathways are still developing and can become permanently altered by traumatic or repeated stress.

We've already been talking about the Fight or Flight response. This doesn't only happen in a real life physical attack, it also happens in an emotional situation/attack. What happens to the body during this time?

Your.....
- pupils dilate to improve vision, awareness intensifies
- heart rate increases
- blood vessels in skin constrict to avoid blood flow in case of injury (responsible for the feeling that your hair is standing on end)
- blood supply increases to muscles, while the systems that are not essential for immediate survival temporarily shut down, i.e. production of saliva reduced (reason why you feel dry mouth)
- breathing speeds up to increase oxygen to the blood
- fat from fat cells and glucose from the liver are metabolized for instant energy
- sweat glands open, providing coolant for overworked system
- Endorphins (natural painkillers) are released

I think you'll easily understand now why the Fight or flight response is not the ideal system for our day to day stresses like unpaid bills or problems at work. It takes a toll on your emotional and physical health. Long term tension, stress, problems can affect your health and manifest as anxiety, chronic worry, anger, hostility, depression, sleep disorders, pain, chronic fatigue, weight gain, low libido, high blood pressure, insulin resistance, autoimmune conditions, etc. The best defense against stress is a healthy lifestyle (incorporating the previous chapters suggestions). Keeping a healthy lifestyle makes you resistant to daily pressures. Don't over extend yourself, don't over promise yourself to people, and don't burn the midnight oil. I cannot stress this enough: it's perfectly OK to tell someone no, turn down an activity, take time for yourself and make yourself a priority. This is your time to get well and letting go of guilt from slowing down could actually be one of the hardest things I'm asking you to do.

Your brain is the central organ of stress. It interprets your environment. It determines your immediate behavioral and physical response to a perceived threat or challenge and your response is based on past experience and what you've learned. The neurocircuitry for social pain actually draws on the neurocircuitry of physical pain so you really do ache when you are lonely or a relationship ends.

Everyone has a different set point for when their stress response is triggered but we can actually change that. Reducing stress can be a highly individualized process. You will need to find what works for the sake of your health.

Relaxation: Your Everyday Right

We have the innate ability to reduce our heart rate, blood pressure and brain wave activity with a "relaxation response". You can achieve many ways such as mediation, yoga, walking, swimming, gardening, anything that takes you out of yourself, but my favorite go-to first step to being more peaceful inside is simple breathing. Research has shown relaxation is effective in treating headaches, premenstrual syndrome, anxiety and mild depression.

. To do the breathing exercises, breathe deeply and count to 8 slowly. HOLD for 8, then release and blow out your mouth for 8. HOLD for 8 and breathe in again to repeat. If you can't do 8 at first, try 5 or even 3 (just don't start doing it fast and hyperventilate instead).   Sometimes when I have a hard time settling in to sleep at night, I use this technique too and it helps me fall asleep.

If you want to check to see if you're doing the breathing right, lying down - lie flat on your back, place a book on your belly, inhale counting 1-5, watch the book rise. hold 1-5. exhale 1-5. hold 1-5.

If you're out or at work, you can do this breathing exercise sitting up too - sit in a straight back chair with feet on the floor. Put your right hand on abdomen (hand should be pushed out by your belly as you inhale and fall as you exhale). Count like above.

If your muscles are tense because of stress or you're stressed because your muscles are tense, it activates your protection and Fight or Flight mode. Tight muscles and tendon fibers stick together and cause pain and this circular problem can increase stress and push us into Fight or Flight mode again. Doing those breathing exercises can help loosen up those muscles. I also sometimes like to use a foam roller to help release tension.

Stress circadian rhythm (our body clock) is largely synchronized by the stress hormone cortisol. When your circadian rhythm is out of whack and you are deprived of sleep, every system in your body undergoes significant physical stress. The National Sleep Foundation says that at least 40 million Americans suffer from sleep disorders. 60% of adults report having problems with sleep including difficulty falling or staying asleep, early waking and interrupted, nonrestorative sleep a few nights a week or more.

Most people think 5-6 hours is fine, but we really need more. As I said in the previous section about detox, 7-8 hours is truly needed, 9-10 would be beneficial for extra detox or times of extra stress. If you need help with sleep, you can try the breathing exercises I mentioned previously while lying in bed, or you could try a supplement called melatonin, or herbs like passionflower, valerian root, ashwagandha, lavender and chamomile tea and make sure your room is dark and free of wifi signals as much as possible.

Before I go into more strategies, I want to mention that if you're not eating right, you're stressing your body whether or not you are under emotional stress. Nutritional deficiency is one of the most powerful stressors. When stressed, you're more vulnerable to nutritional deficiencies. Then your body's response to deficiencies increases stress. We need the absolute best nutrition when under stress. When you eat better you become "stress-resilient". With good nutrition, you can improve your mood, have more stamina and vitality and prevent disease.

Reframing and Neutralizing Stress: Getting Your Mind to Work for Your Body

Your mind is constantly screening situations. It assesses if a situation is harmful, threatening, challenging or helpful. Stress is not because of a situation or a person. It is the interaction of the person with a situation. A person in a stressful situation creates their stress reaction. The way you perceive a particular situation determines whether or not it is stressful for you. Stress can motivate you, make you alert and productive and give you vitality. Your response (your emotional, behavioral, and physical reactions) results from a mental judgement you've made. You judge something as a threat or you think you can cope with it and your response to stress is a product of your past experience, personality, lifestyle, and culture.

Situations can cause stress because:
- The more important the goal, the more intense the emotion
- The situation threatens what you want and makes you frustrated
- Something important to you is being threatened: self-esteem, positive opinion of others, your ideals, moral values, or beliefs, people you love or objects you value

- You blame yourself or others for a bad situation. If you take the blame, you will experience guilt, shame, and anger at yourself. If you blame others, you'll be angry.
- You think things won't work out in your favor. Having expectations that your situation will turn out badly results in negative emotions.
- The demands of a situation exceed your ability to cope with it
- Your appraisal of the situation is inaccurate because you overestimate what the situation demands or you underestimate your ability to cope. Feeling powerless or overwhelmed leads to stress.
- You exaggerate the consequences of not being able to cope
- Expectations, beliefs or fears keep you from using your coping skills
- You lack an adequate support system or fears keep you from using your support system

Emotions that can trigger physical stress depending on severity – anger, anxiety, fear, guilt, shame, sadness, grief, envy, jealousy

People who tend to live on high stress mode are generally more intense and are prone to anger, anxiety, envy, jealousy, and optimism, while more laid back stress responders are more likely to turn inward in sadness, fear, guilt, shame, hopelessness and pessimism. You can also create stress simply by anticipating a stressful situation. These are the people that think about what might happen IF…… and sadly, I'm one of those overthinkers.

Let's use that now to see just how we can reframe and neutralize our stressors. (see appendix for blank sheet)

Trigger - Write down an event or situation that has triggered or is triggering stress	Record the thoughts that are going through your head or have gone through your head	Consequence List the feelings you are experiencing or have experienced
You are not asked to a social event with your friends	Being left out is a disaster I'm not important enough My friends must not like me that much I don't measure up	Anxiety Shame Fear Worry

Now you can learn some mindful restructuring to de-stress this situation.

1. Become aware of harmful core beliefs and negative thought patterns
2. Challenge the stress inducing mindsets
3. Replace them with healthy, affirming, balanced thoughts and beliefs

The idea is to dispute our knee jerk reaction thoughts and replace them with a positive alternative to an automatic negative thought. Then we are going to Energize with effective new approaches. Once you get used to thinking in this way, your knee jerk reaction will change and be replaced with non-stressful new approaches and thoughts.

Diffusing thought/question	Positive substitution
Does everyone always attend all gatherings? There are enough get-togethers that missing one is not a crisis Not being included does not necessarily reflect your friend's opinion of you	View not having to go as found time to relax and pamper yourself Ask your friend if you can go to the gathering (maybe it was an unintentional oversight)

When you are in a stressful situation, ask yourself these questions:

- How do I feel?
- What am I thinking?
- What core beliefs are influencing my perception of what happened?
- Are any cognitive distortions contributing to my stressful response?
- Do my assumptions accurately reflect what happened?
- Do the facts support my interpretation?
- Is there a more positive way to interpret the event?
- If I'm right, what is the worst that can happen?
- Am I understanding my ability to handle the consequences of the event?
- What can I do to improve the situation?

Use this sheet in the appendix throughout the week each time you feel something is bothering you, big or small. When you get into the habit enough, you won't need the sheet and your mind will be retrained to think differently (your knee jerk reaction will change) and your body will react more calmly too. Your physical and mental health will benefit from changing your thoughts in this way.

The last technique I want to talk to you about today is called Emotional Freedom Technique which is also called tapping.

Tapping: Clearing Your Body's Short Circuits

Tapping, also known as Emotional Freedom Technique (EFT) has its history in Chinese medicine. It's somewhat similar in concept to acupuncture, but you don't have to be jabbed with needles. It's a psychological acupressure technique where you just use your own fingers. The basis is that you need to clear your body's meridians or energy fields of negativity. Gary Craig brought EFT to the forefront in 1995 and he said, "The cause of all negative emotions is a disruption in the body's Energy System."

When you use tapping through the energy meridians and voicing positive affirmation, it works to clear the "short-circuit" (the emotional block) from your body's bioenergy system. It restores your mind and body's balance, which is essential for wellness and the resolution of physical illness and symptoms.

Tapping is pretty simple to do, but one session may not clear your issues. During tapping, you will be doing 2 things – tapping and saying positive affirmations. Note: it's best to do this without glasses on because it can mess with the electromagnetics.

Here are the steps:
1. Define the negative emotion. Give it a number 1-10 (10 being high severity)
2. Use a clarifying phrase. "Even though I have _____, I totally and completely love, forgive

and accept myself anyway" or the 2nd half can be "I totally and completely accept myself" or "I totally and completely love and accept myself".

3. Repeat the clarifying phrase and tap the karate chop point.
4. Use a reminder phrase for all the other points
5. Tap through all the points repeating the phrase

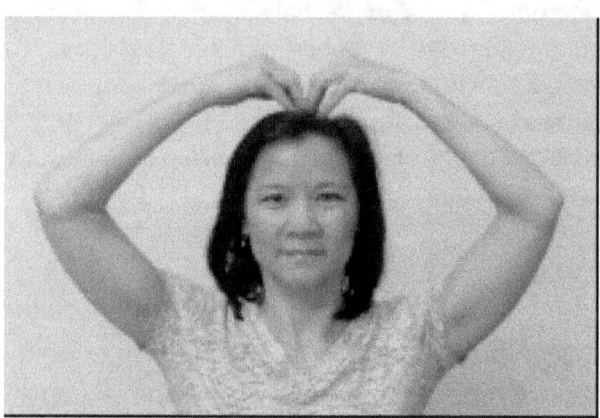

1. Top of the Head (TH)
With fingers back-to-back down the center of the skull.

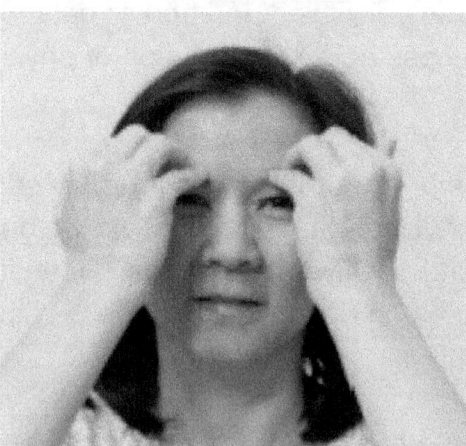

2. Eyebrow (EB)
Just above and to one side of the nose, at the beginning of the eyebrow.

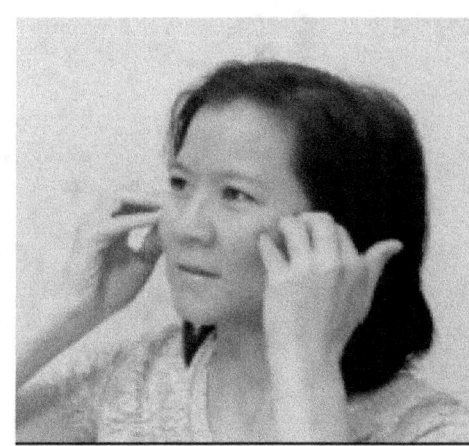

3. Side of the Eye (SE)
On the bone bordering the outside corner of the eye.

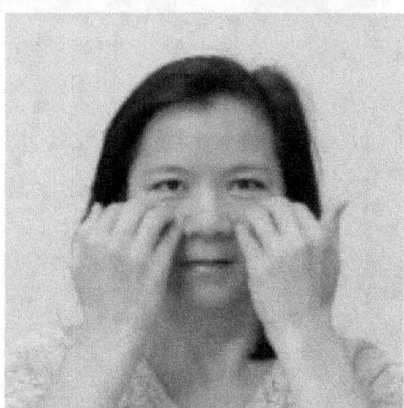

4. Under the Eye (UE)
On the bone under an eye about 1 inch below your pupil.

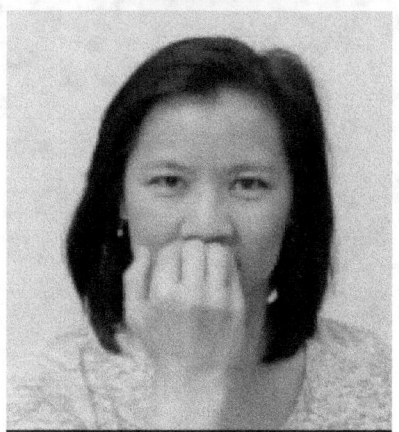

5. Under the Nose (UN)
On the small area between the bottom of your nose and the top of your upper lip.

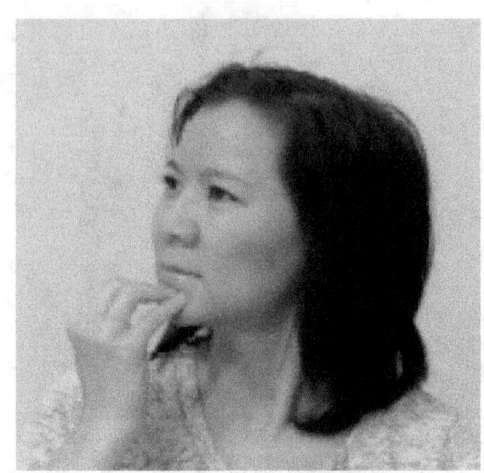

6. Chin (Ch)

Midway between the point of your chin and the bottom of your lower lip. Even though it is not directly on the point of the chin, we call it the chin point because it is descriptive enough for people to understand easily.

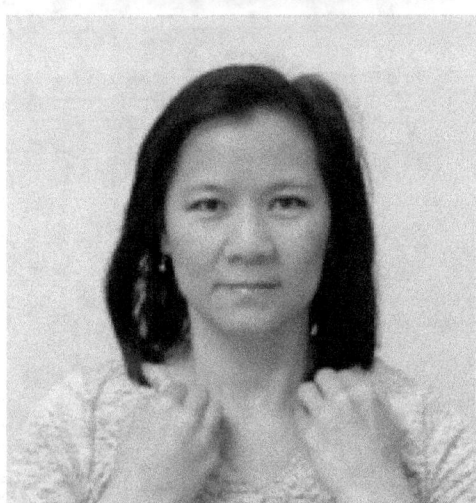

7. Collar Bone (CB)

The junction where the sternum (breastbone), collarbone and the first rib meet. This is a very important point and in acupuncture is referred to as K (kidney) 27. To locate it, first place your forefinger on the U-shaped notch at the top of the breastbone (about where a man would knot his tie). From the bottom of the U, move your forefinger down toward the navel 1 inch and then go to the left (or right) 1 inch. This point is referred to as Collar Bone even though it is not on the collarbone (or clavicle) per se.

8. Under the Arm (UA)

On the side of the body, at a point even with the nipple (for men) or in the middle of the bra strap (for women). It is about 4 inches below the armpit.

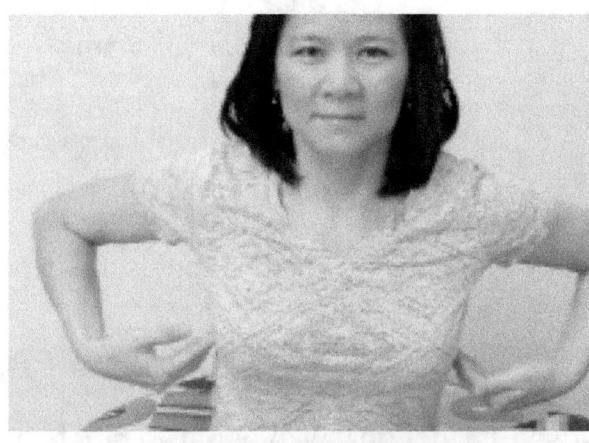

9. Wrists (WR)

The last point is the inside of both wrists.

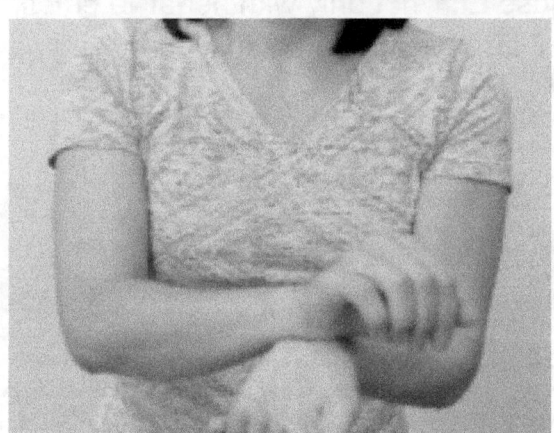

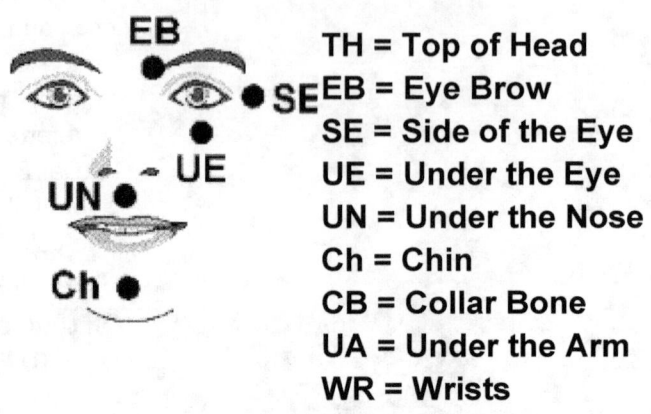

TH = Top of Head
EB = Eye Brow
SE = Side of the Eye
UE = Under the Eye
UN = Under the Nose
Ch = Chin
CB = Collar Bone
UA = Under the Arm
WR = Wrists

Per Dr. Mercola http://eft.mercola.com/

6. Ask yourself what severity your issue is now. Assign it a number again.

7. Repeat until your severity is 2 or lower.

You can use EFT not only with negative emotions (past and present), but also with food cravings, reducing pain or to implement positive goals.

Maintenance for Everyday Wellness

I find that having rituals makes my life peaceful. Knowing exactly how each day starts and ends helps me to have less stress and it helps me do the right things for my body.

I find that people try to put too much into their morning ritual. Morning rituals should not be things you have to kick yourself into gear to do – like exercising. It should be something you look forward to when you get up and should not take longer than 30 minutes.

In the beginning it may be hard, but after about 30 days you'll be doing these rituals like it's second nature.

Your morning rituals will be different that everyone else's but ideas are:

- Drinking water first thing
- Bathroom hygiene and time on the toilet (yes, I'm serious!)
- Detox drink
- Simple Stretches
- Bath or shower
- Review schedule and goals for the day

The benefit of the morning ritual is to give you a positive point to start from each day. If you feel you need something to get you in a good mood, maybe find something funny or inspiring on youtube and watch different things start your day in a good mood.

While having a morning ritual is important to starting off the day and really getting the most out of it, an evening ritual is almost equally as important as it really allows you to absorb everything that happened that day, wind down from the day and review what is scheduled (or not scheduled for tomorrow).

One of the hardest things to help keep your positive outlook is to celebrate the little things and successes that you may have had during the day. We all tend to want every second to be good and every day to be "productive" before we'll look back on the day and say it was good. Instead, try looking back on the day (reframing it) and celebrate what you were able to do and look at things in a positive light. Don't beat yourself up for not finishing something, being unable to do something or feeling like you've let yourself or someone else down.

Ideas for evening rituals:
- Soak in the bath (Epsom salt, baking soda, hydrogen peroxide)
- Detox Tea
- Sleep Tea
- Alone time for yourself/meditation
- Relaxing book or movie
- Gentle stretching
- Turn off electronics
- Journaling

I generally unwind with TV in my bedroom for a while, write my schedule for the day (or review it on my phone), try to clear my mind, do some self massage or lymph drainage if needed, stretch out sore joints and I may use my infrared heating pad for aches and pains. I notice when I don't have this downtime before sleep, it takes me longer to get to sleep, I don't sleep as deeply and life becomes more stressful each day I miss my time to myself.

Afterwards

A last note on friends:

I talk to a lot of people who now because of their health are unable to go out and do things. Some of those friends can be very negative and this is not good for your health. You may need to be more proactive about who you surround yourself and release your guilt about who you choose to stay around.

It's really okay to get a new circle of friends. Life comes in stages and friends do come and go. If you look back in life there were friends that came in and friends that went out. IT'S OK! You can end or put on hold the relationships that you've been trying to save with people who stopped calling and caring when you got sick.

This is your only life. If you are unwell it's up to you to decide on the relationships and environmental factors that you can control. Besides, stressful friendships (or family) cause flare ups.

If you feel like you have no one, find facebook groups. I spent so many days with my online friends being way more supportive as strangers than those I had known for years. They understand if they're in the same boat. It is possible to have meaningful friendships despite health issues and chronic illness. You can have meaning without DOING more or giving more than you are able.

It's okay to switch friends. Let go of toxic friends so you can heal. You haven't turned your back on those other friends – you're no turncoat, you just need to have the support you deserve to get through your health journey. I have made so many great online friends and some I would say now are better friends than the friends I know in person. I have no regrets in switching friends – it's been just what I needed to help me heal.

Appendix

Reframing Stress

Trigger (situation that activated stress)	Self-Talk (thoughts that go through your head)	Consequences (feelings you experience)	Diffusing Questions or Thoughts	Positive Substitution (positive alternative to negative thought)

McClelland, Stephanie M.D. and Hamilton, Beth Hamilton M.D. *So Stressed: The Ultimate Stress-Relief for Women* New York: Atria Books, 2009. Print